The New Menopause Cookbook for Beginners

Simple and Nourishing Recipes for a Healthy Menopause Transition

I0766450

copyrighted@2024

Jennifer Monet

Table of Contents

Chapter One

The New Menopause Cookbook

Introduction

Understanding Menopause and the Power of Food

Menopause is a significant transition in a woman's life that usually occurs between the ages of 45 and 55. This phase brings various physical and emotional changes due to hormonal changes. The right diet can help manage symptoms, promote overall health and improve well-being. This cookbook offers a collection of delicious and nutritious recipes designed to address the unique needs of women during menopause.

Menopause Transition and Nutrition

The Role of Diet in Menopause

Menopause is a significant biological event that marks the end of a woman's menstrual cycle and reproductive years. This phase is officially diagnosed after 12 consecutive months without menstruation and usually occurs between the ages of 45 and 55. During this transition, substantial hormonal changes occur in the body, primarily a drop in estrogen

and progesterone levels, which
can lead to various symptoms
and health risks.

Hormonal Changes and Symptoms

Hot flashes and night sweats:
Sudden feelings of warmth in the
upper body that can lead to
sweating and discomfort.

Mood swings: Fluctuations in
hormone levels can affect
neurotransmitters in the brain,
leading to mood swings,
irritability, and even depression.

Sleep disorders: Hormonal
changes can disrupt sleep

patterns and cause insomnia or disturbed sleep.

Weight gain: Metabolism slows down and fat distribution may change, especially in the abdominal area.

Loss of bone density: Decreased estrogen levels can lead to decreased bone density, increasing the risk of osteoporosis.

Cardiovascular health: The risk of heart disease may increase due to changes in cholesterol levels and blood vessel health.

Vaginal dryness: Decreased estrogen can cause vaginal

tissues to thin and dry, leading to discomfort.

Nutritional Needs

During menopause, certain nutrients are especially important to help manage symptoms and promote overall health. Here are the main nutrients to focus on:

Key nutrients for menopause

1. Calcium and vitamin D

Why: Essential for bone health; calcium supports bone density and vitamin D aids calcium absorption.

Sources: Leafy greens, almonds, fortified dairy or plant-based milk,

and fatty fish for calcium.
Sunlight and foods fortified with
vitamin D.

Tips: Aim for at least 1,200 mg of
calcium and 600,800 IU of
vitamin D per day. If your diet is
insufficient, consider taking
supplements.

2. Omega3 fatty acids

Why: Reduces inflammation,
supports heart health, and can
moderate mood swings.

Sources: Fatty fish (salmon,
mackerel, sardines), flax seeds,
chia seeds and walnuts.

Tips: Include fatty fish in your diet at least twice a week or consider omega3 supplements.

3. Phytoestrogens

Why: Plant compounds that can mimic estrogen in the body and help ease menopausal symptoms.

Sources: Soy products (tofu, tempeh, edamame), flaxseeds and legumes.

Tips: Include these foods regularly to help balance your hormone levels.

4. Fiber

Why: Supports digestion, helps manage weight and regulates blood sugar.

Sources: Whole grains, fruits, vegetables and legumes.

Tips: Aim for at least 25 grams of fiber a day.

5. Antioxidants

Why: Fight oxidative stress and promote overall health.

Sources: Berries, nuts, seeds and colorful vegetables.

Tips: Consume a variety of colorful fruits and veggies every day.

6. Magnesium

Why: Helps with muscle function, sleep and bone health.

Sources: Nuts, seeds, whole grains, and leafy greens.

Tips: Consider magnesium supplements if dietary intake is insufficient, especially if you experience muscle cramps or sleep disturbances.

Building a Menopause-Friendly Kitchen

Stocking your kitchen with the right ingredients and tools is essential to making healthy eating easier. Here are some tips:

Basic ingredients:

Whole grains: Brown rice, quinoa, oats, and whole grain bread.

Lean proteins: chicken, turkey, tofu, tempeh, beans and legumes.

Healthy fats: Olive oil, avocado, almonds, seeds, and oily fish.

Fruits and vegetables: Various color options, fresh and frozen.

Dairy products or alternatives: Low-fat dairy products, fortified plant-based milks and yogurts.

Spices and herbs: Turmeric, ginger, garlic, basil and oregano for flavor and health benefits.

Kitchen tools:

Quality cookware: Invest in non-stick pans, sturdy pans and baking trays.

Blender / food processor: For smoothies, soups and healthy snacks.

Storage Containers: Keep your fridge and pantry organized with airtight food prep containers.

Slow Cooker / Instant Pot: For convenient and nutritious one-pot meals.

Chapter Two

Breakfast Recipes

Energizing Breakfast Ideas

Start your day with a nutritious breakfast that can set the tone for the rest of your day. These breakfast recipes are designed to provide essential nutrients, boost energy levels and help manage menopause symptoms.

1. Chia Seed Pudding with Berries

Ingredients:

3 tablespoons of chia seeds

1 cup almond milk (or other preferred milk)

1 tablespoon of honey or maple syrup

1/2 teaspoon of vanilla extract

1/2 cup mixed fruit (strawberries, blueberries, raspberries)

Instruction:

1. Mix chia seeds, almond milk, honey and vanilla extract in a bowl.

2. Mix well to combine and let sit for about 10 minutes. Stir again to prevent clumping.

3. Cover and refrigerate overnight.

4. Mix well in the morning and put the blended berries on top.

5. Eat chilled.

2. Spinach and Feta Omelet

Ingredients:

2 large eggs

1/4 cup chopped spinach

2 tablespoons of crumbled feta cheese

1 teaspoon of olive oil

Salt and pepper to taste

Instruction:

1. In a bowl, beat the eggs with a pinch of salt and pepper.

2. In a nonstick frying pan, heat the olive oil over medium.

3. Add chopped spinach and sauté until wilted.

4. Pour the beaten eggs over the spinach and cook until the eggs are almost set.

5. Sprinkle half of the omelette with feta cheese.

6. Fold the omelet in half and cook for another minute.

7. Serve warm.

3. Quinoa Breakfast Bowl

Ingredients:

1 cup cooked quinoa

1/2 cup almond milk

1 banana, sliced

1/4 cup walnuts, chopped

1/2 teaspoon ground cinnamon

1 tablespoon honey or maple syrup (optional)

Instruction:

1. Heat the cooked quinoa in a small saucepan with the almond milk over low heat.

2. Stir in ground cinnamon and honey or maple syrup, if using.

3. Transfer to a bowl and top with banana slices and chopped walnuts.

4. Serve warm.

4. Greek yogurt parfait

Ingredients:

1 cup Greek yogurt

1/2 cup granola

1/2 cup mixed berries (blueberries, raspberries, strawberries)

1 tablespoon of honey or maple syrup

1 tablespoon of flax seeds

Instruction:

1. Layer half of the Greek yogurt in a glass or bowl.

2. Top with granola and mixed berries.

3. Top with remaining Greek yogurt.

4. Drizzle with honey or maple syrup.

5. Sprinkle with flax seeds and serve immediately.

5. Avocado Toast with Poached Egg

Ingredients:

1 slice whole wheat bread, toasted

1/2 ripe avocado

1 fried egg

Salt and pepper to taste

Red pepper flakes (optional)

Lemon juice (optional)

Instruction:

1. Mash the avocado in a bowl
with a fork. Add salt, pepper and
a squeeze of lemon juice if
needed.

2. Spread the mashed avocado on
the toasted bread.

3. Put a fried egg on top.

4. Sprinkle with red pepper flakes
for an extra kick.

5. Serve immediately.

6. Berry Smoothie Bowl

Ingredients:

1 cup frozen mixed berries

1 banana

1/2 cup almond milk

1/2 cup Greek yogurt

1 teaspoon of chia seeds

1/4 cup granola (for topping)

1 tablespoon grated coconut (for topping)

Instruction:

1. Combine frozen berries, banana, almond milk, Greek

yogurt and chia seeds in a
blender. Blend until smooth.

2. Pour the smoothie into a bowl.

3. Top with granola and grated
coconut.

4. Serve immediately with a
spoon.

Chapter Three

Lunch Recipes

Hearty and Nutritious Lunches

A nutritious lunch can provide the energy and nutrients you need to get you through the day, especially during menopause. These recipes are designed to be delicious and beneficial for managing menopause symptoms and promoting overall health.

1. Grilled Chicken and Avocado Salad

Ingredients:

1 grilled chicken breast, cut into slices

4 cups mixed greens (spinach, arugula, kale)

1 avocado, sliced

1/2 cup cherry tomatoes, halved

1/4 cup red onion, thinly sliced

2 tablespoons of olive oil

1 tablespoon of lemon juice

Salt and pepper to taste

Instruction:

1. Combine mixed greens, cherry tomatoes and red onion in a large bowl.

2. Top with sliced grilled chicken and avocado.

3. Whisk olive oil, lemon juice, salt and pepper in a small bowl.

4. Drizzle the dressing over the salad and gently toss.

5. Serve immediately.

2. Lentil and Vegetable Soup

Ingredients:

1 cup dried lentils, rinsed

1 carrot, diced

2 stalks of celery, diced

1 onion, chopped

2 cloves of garlic, chopped

1 can (14.5 oz) diced tomatoes

4 cups of vegetable broth

1 teaspoon of dried thyme

1 teaspoon dried basil

1 bay leaf

Salt and pepper to taste

2 cups spinach, roughly chopped

Instruction:

1. In a large pot, sauté onion, carrot, and celery over medium heat until softened, about 5 minutes.

2. Add the garlic and simmer for another minute.

3. Stir in the lentils, chopped tomatoes, vegetable stock, thyme, basil and bay leaf.

4. Bring to a boil, reduce the heat and cook for 3035 minutes until the lentils are tender.

5. Add salt and pepper to taste.

6. Add the chopped spinach and simmer for about 2 minutes, or until wilted.

7. Remove the bay leaf and serve hot.

3. Tofu Stir-Fry

Ingredients:

1 block of firm tofu, drained and diced

1 red pepper, sliced

1 yellow bell pepper, sliced

1 cup broccoli florets

1 carrot, julienned

2 spoons of soy sauce

1 tablespoon of olive oil

1 tablespoon of sesame oil

2 cloves of garlic, chopped

1 teaspoon grated ginger

2 tablespoons of water

1 teaspoon cornstarch

Instruction:

1. Heat olive oil in a large skillet or wok over medium-high heat.

2. Add tofu cubes and fry until golden on all sides, about 57

minutes. Remove from pan and set aside.

3. In the same pan, add the sesame oil and sauté the garlic and ginger until fragrant, about 1 minute.

4. Add peppers, broccoli and carrots. Cook the vegetables for about 5 minutes, until they are soft.

5. In a small bowl, mix the soy sauce, water and cornstarch. Pour into the pan and toss to coat the vegetables.

6. Add the tofu back to the pan and stir.

7. Serve hot with brown rice or quinoa.

4. Quinoa and Black Beans Stuffed Peppers

Ingredients:

4 peppers (any color), cut off the tops and remove the seeds

1 cup cooked quinoa

1 can (15 ounces) of black beans, washed and drained

1 cup corn kernels (fresh or frozen)

1/2 cup chopped tomatoes

1/2 cup grated cheddar cheese (optional)

1 teaspoon cumin

1 teaspoon of chili powder

Salt and pepper to taste

Fresh cilantro, chopped (for garnish)

Instruction:

1. Preheat oven to 375°F (190°C).

2. In a large bowl, combine the cooked quinoa, black beans, corn, diced tomatoes, cumin, chili powder, salt, and pepper.

3. Stuff each pepper with the quinoa mixture.

4. Place the stuffed peppers in the baking dish and cover with aluminum foil.

5. Bake for 30 minutes. If using cheese, remove the foil, sprinkle with cheese and bake for a further 10 minutes until the cheese has melted and the pepper has softened.

6. Garnish with fresh cilantro before serving.

5. Mediterranean Chickpea Salad

Ingredients:

1 can (15 ounces) of drained and rinsed chickpeas

1 cucumber, diced

1 cup cherry tomatoes, halved

1/4 red onion, thinly sliced

1/4 cup Kalamata olives, pitted
and sliced

1/4 cup feta cheese, crumbled

2 tablespoons of olive oil

1 tablespoon red wine vinegar

1 teaspoon of dried oregano

Salt and pepper to taste

Instruction:

1. In a large bowl, combine the
chickpeas, cucumber, cherry

tomatoes, red onion, olives and feta cheese.

2. In a small bowl, mix olive oil, red wine vinegar, oregano, salt and pepper.

3. Toss the salad with the dressing until well combined.

4. Serve chilled or at room temperature.

6. Sweet Potato Black Bean Burrito Bowl

Ingredients:

1 large sweet potato, peeled and diced

1 can (15 ounces) of black beans, washed and drained

1 cup cooked brown rice

1 avocado, sliced

1/2 cup salsa

1/4 cup Greek yogurt

1 tablespoon of olive oil

1 teaspoon cumin

1/2 teaspoon chili powder

Salt and pepper to taste

Instruction:

1. Preheat oven to 400°F (200°C).

2. Mix diced sweet potatoes with olive oil, cumin, chili, salt and pepper. Spread on a baking sheet

and bake for 2025 minutes until soft.

3. Layer brown rice, black beans and roasted sweet potatoes in a bowl.

4. Top with slices of avocado, salsa and a dollop of Greek yogurt.

5. Serve immediately.

Chapter Four

Dinner Recipes

Delicious and Balanced Dinners

A well-balanced dinner can help you wind down after a long day and ensure you get the nutrients you need to support your health during menopause. These recipes are designed to be delicious and beneficial for managing menopause symptoms and promoting overall well-being.

1. Baked Salmon with Quinoa and Asparagus

Ingredients:

2 salmon fillets

1 cup quinoa, rinsed

2 cups of water or vegetable broth

1 bunch asparagus, chopped

2 tablespoons of olive oil

1 lemon, cut into slices

2 cloves of garlic, chopped

Salt and pepper to taste

Fresh dill, chopped (for garnish)

Instruction:

1. Preheat oven to 400°F (200°C).

2. Place the salmon fillets on a baking sheet lined with baking paper. Drizzle 1 tablespoon of olive oil, season with salt, pepper and crushed garlic. Top with lemon slices.

3. Arrange the asparagus around the salmon, drizzle with the remaining olive oil and season with salt and pepper.

4. Bake for 1520 minutes until the salmon is cooked and the asparagus is tender.

5. Meanwhile, bring water or vegetable stock to a boil in a medium saucepan. Add the quinoa, reduce the heat to low,

cover and cook for 15 minutes until the quinoa is cooked.

6. Fluff the quinoa with a fork and serve with roasted salmon and asparagus. Garnish with fresh dill.

2. Spaghetti Squash with Tomato Basil Sauce

Ingredients:

1 large spaghetti squash

2 tablespoons of olive oil

1 onion, chopped

3 cloves of garlic, chopped

1 can (28 ounces) crushed tomatoes

1/2 teaspoon dried oregano

1/2 teaspoon dried basil

Salt and pepper to taste

1/4 cup fresh basil, chopped

Grated Parmesan (optional)

Instruction:

1. Preheat oven to 400°F (200°C).

2. Cut the spaghetti squash in half lengthwise, then scrape out the seeds. Place cut side down on a baking sheet and bake for 4045 minutes until tender.

3. While the pumpkin is baking, heat the olive oil in a large skillet over medium heat. Sauté the onion and garlic until soft.

4. Add the smashed tomatoes, oregano, basil, salt, and pepper. Cook for 1520 minutes.

5. Once the pumpkin is done, use a fork to scrape the spaghetti strands into a bowl.

6. Serve spaghetti squash topped with tomato basil sauce and garnish with fresh basil and Parmesan cheese to taste.

3. Chickpea and Spinach Curry

Ingredients:

1 can (15 ounces) of drained and rinsed chickpeas

2 cups spinach, roughly chopped

1 onion, chopped

3 cloves of garlic, chopped

1 tablespoon ginger, grated

1 can (14 ounces) coconut milk

1 can (14.5 oz) diced tomatoes

2 spoons of curry

1 tablespoon of olive oil

Salt and pepper to taste

Fresh cilantro, chopped (for garnish)

Cooked Brown Rice (to serve)

Instruction:

1. In a large skillet, heat the olive oil over medium heat. Fry the

onion, garlic and ginger until fragrant.

2. Add the curry and cook for another minute.

3. Stir in chickpeas, chopped tomatoes and coconut milk. Cook for 1520 minutes until the sauce thickens.

4. Add the chopped spinach and simmer until wilted.

5. Add salt and pepper to taste.

6. Serve with cooked brown rice and garnish with fresh cilantro.

4. Turkey and Vegetable Stuffed Peppers

Ingredients:

4 peppers (any color), cut off the tops and remove the seeds

1 pound ground turkey

1 cup cooked brown rice

1 zucchini, diced

1 carrot, diced

1 onion, chopped

2 cloves of garlic, chopped

1 can (14.5 oz) diced tomatoes

1 tablespoon of olive oil

1 teaspoon of dried oregano

1 teaspoon dried basil

Salt and pepper to taste

1/2 cup shredded mozzarella cheese (optional)

Instruction:

1. Preheat oven to 375°F (190°C).

2. Heat the olive oil in a big skillet over medium heat. Sauté the onion and garlic until soft.

3. Add ground turkey and cook until browned. Stir in diced zucchini, carrots and tomatoes.

4. Season with oregano, basil, salt and pepper. Cook until the vegetables are soft.

5. Stir in the cooked brown rice.

6. Stuff each pepper with the turkey and vegetable mixture.

7. Place the stuffed peppers in a baking dish and cover with aluminum foil. Bake for 30 minutes.

8. If using cheese, remove the foil, sprinkle with cheese and bake for a further 10 minutes until the cheese has melted and the pepper has softened.

9. Serve hot.

5. Shrimp and Broccoli Stir-Fry

Ingredients:

1 pound shrimp, peeled and deveined

2 cups broccoli florets

1 red pepper, sliced

2 spoons of soy sauce

1 tablespoon oyster sauce

1 tablespoon of olive oil

2 cloves of garlic, chopped

1 teaspoon grated ginger

Mix 1 teaspoon cornstarch with 2 tablespoons of water.

Boiled jasmine rice (for serving)

Sesame seeds (for garnishing)

Instruction:

1. Heat olive oil in a large skillet
or wok over medium-high heat.
Cook until the garlic and ginger
are fragrant.

2. Add shrimp and cook until
pink, about 34 minutes. Remove
from pan and set aside.

3. Add the broccoli and peppers
to the same pan. Cook until
tender, about 5 minutes.

4. Stir in soy sauce, oyster sauce
and cornstarch mixture. Cook
until the sauce thickens.

5. Add the shrimp back to the pan
and toss to coat with the sauce.

6. Serve with steamed jasmine rice and garnish with sesame seeds.

6. Eggplant Parmesan

Ingredients:

2 large eggplants cut into 1/2-inch rounds

1 cup whole wheat breadcrumbs

1/2 cup grated parmesan

2 eggs, beaten

2 cups marinara sauce

1 cup of grated mozzarella cheese

1 tablespoon of olive oil

Fresh basil, chopped (for garnish)

Instruction:

1. Preheat oven to 375°F (190°C).

2. Dip the eggplant slices in beaten eggs, then cover with a mixture of breadcrumbs and Parmesan cheese.

3. In a large skillet set over medium heat, heat the olive oil. Frying the eggplant slices on each sides until golden.

4. Spread a layer of marinara sauce into the baking dish. Top with eggplant slices, then top with more marinara sauce and shredded mozzarella cheese.

5. Repeat the layers until all the ingredients are used up, ending with a layer of cheese.

6. Bake for 2530 minutes until the cheese has melted and risen.

7. Garnish with fresh basil before serving.

Snack and Smoothie Recipes

Nutritious and Tasty Snacks and Smoothies

Snacking can be a healthy way to maintain energy levels and curb hunger between meals. These snack and smoothie recipes are designed to be nutritious and support your menopause health, providing essential vitamins, minerals and antioxidants.

Snacks

1. Almond and Berry Yogurt Parfait

Ingredients:

1 cup Greek yogurt

1/4 cup fresh or frozen mixed berries

2 tablespoons of grated almonds

1 tablespoon of honey or maple syrup

Instruction:

1. In a bowl or glass, layer Greek yogurt, mixed berries and chopped almonds.

2. Drizzle with honey or maple syrup.

3. Enjoy immediately or refrigerate for later.

2. Hummus and Veggie Sticks

Ingredients:

1 cup hummus

1 carrot, cut into sticks

1 cucumber, cut into sticks

1 red pepper, cut into sticks

1 stalk of celery, cut into sticks

Instruction:

1. Arrange the vegetable sticks on a plate.

2. Serve with a bowl of hummus for dipping.

3. Apple Slices with Nut Butter

Ingredients:

1 apple, sliced

2 tablespoons almond or peanut butter

1 tablespoon chia seeds (optional)

Instruction:

1. Spread the apple slices with nut butter.

2. Sprinkle with chia seeds as needed for added crunch and nutrition.

3. Enjoy immediately.

Smoothies

1. Green Detox Smoothie

Ingredients:

1 cup spinach

1 banana

1/2 cup cucumber, sliced

1/2 cup pineapple chunks (fresh or frozen)

1 cup coconut water

1 teaspoon of chia seeds

Instruction:

1. Blend all of the ingredients.

2. Blend until smooth.

3. Serve immediately.

2. Berry Blast Smoothie

Ingredients:

1 cup mixed fruit (blueberries, raspberries, strawberries)

1 banana

1 cup almond milk

1/2 cup Greek yogurt

1 tablespoon honey or maple syrup (optional)

Instruction:

1. Blend all of the ingredients.

2. Blend until smooth.

3. Serve immediately.

3. Tropical Mango Smoothie

Ingredients:

1 cup mango chunks (fresh or frozen)

1/2 cup pineapple chunks (fresh or frozen)

1 banana

1 cup orange juice

1/2 cup coconut milk

Instruction:

1. Mix all the ingredients in a blender.

2. Blend until smooth.

3. Serve immediately.

Chapter Five

Desserts

Sweet Treats for Menopause Wellness

Indulging in sweet treats doesn't have to derail your health goals. These dessert recipes are designed to satisfy your sweet tooth while providing beneficial nutrients that support your health during menopause.

1. Dark Chocolate Almond Bark

Ingredients:

1 cup dark chocolate (70% cocoa or more)

1/2 cup almonds, chopped

1/4 cup dried cranberries

1/4 cup pumpkin seeds

Sea salt, for sprinkling

Instruction:

1. In a microwave-safe bowl, melt the dark chocolate chips, stirring every 30 seconds, until they are smooth.

2. Stir in chopped almonds, dried cranberries and pumpkin seeds.

3. Pour the mixture onto a tray lined with baking paper and spread evenly.

4. Sprinkle with sea salt.

5. Refrigerate for at least 30 minutes until the chocolate hardens.

6. Break into pieces and store in an airtight container in the refrigerator.

2. Chia Seed Pudding

Ingredients:

1/4 cup chia seeds

1 cup almond milk

1 tablespoon of honey or maple syrup

1/2 teaspoon of vanilla extract

Fresh strawberries, for topping

Instruction:

1. Whisk chia seeds, almond milk, honey and vanilla extract in a bowl.

2. Refrigerate for at least 4 hours, preferably overnight, stirring occasionally.

3. Before serving, mix well and garnish with fresh fruit.

3. Baked Apples with Cinnamon and Walnuts

Ingredients:

4 cored apples

1/4 cup walnuts, chopped

2 tablespoons of honey or maple syrup

1 teaspoon ground cinnamon

1/2 teaspoon ground nutmeg

Instruction:

1. Preheat oven to 350°F
(175°C).

2. Place the cored apples in the
baking dish.

3. In a small bowl, mix the
walnuts, honey, cinnamon and
nutmeg.

4. Fill each apple with the nut
mixture.

5. Bake for 2530 minutes until
the apples are soft.

6. Serve warm.

4. Greek Yogurt with Honey and Pistachios

Ingredients:

1 cup Greek yogurt

2 spoons of honey

2 tablespoons pistachios, chopped

1/2 teaspoon ground cinnamon

Instruction:

1. Pour a spoonful of Greek yogurt into a serving bowl.

2. Drizzle with honey.

3. Sprinkle with chopped pistachios and ground cinnamon.

4. Serve immediately.

5. Avocado Chocolate Mousse

Ingredients:

2 ripe avocados

1/4 cup cocoa powder

1/4 cup honey or maple syrup

1/4 cup almond milk

1 teaspoon of vanilla extract

Fresh berries or nuts for topping
(optional)

Instruction:

1. Blend avocado, cocoa powder,
honey, almond milk and vanilla
extract in a food processor until
smooth and creamy.

2. Spoon the mousse into serving bowls.

3. Place in the refrigerator for at least 30 minutes before serving.

4. Add fresh fruit or nuts if desired.

Beverages

Refreshing and Nutritious Drinks

Staying hydrated and enjoying healthy beverages is essential for overall well-being, especially during menopause. These drink recipes are designed to be refreshing and nutritious, providing hydration along with beneficial nutrients.

1. Herbal Iced Tea

Ingredients:

4 cups of water

4 herbal tea bags (such as chamomile, peppermint or hibiscus)

1 tablespoon honey or maple syrup (optional)

Fresh mint leaves (for garnish)

Lemon slices (for garnish)

Instruction:

1. Boil the water and pour the tea bags in a heatproof jug.

2. Leave to steep for 510 minutes, then remove the tea bags.

3. Stir in honey or maple syrup as needed.

4. Allow the tea to come to room temperature before chilling.

5. Serve over ice, topped with fresh mint leaves and lemon slices.

2. Golden Milk (Turmeric Latte)

Ingredients:

2 cups almond milk (or any other plant-based milk).

1 teaspoon ground turmeric

1/2 teaspoon ground cinnamon

1/2 teaspoon ground ginger

1 tablespoon of honey or maple syrup

1/2 teaspoon of vanilla extract

A pinch of black pepper

Instruction:

1. In a small saucepan, combine the almond milk, turmeric, cinnamon, ginger, honey, vanilla extract, and black pepper.

2. Heat over medium heat, whisking constantly, until warm and well combined.

3. Pour into mugs and serve warm.

3. Green Smoothie

Ingredients:

1 cup spinach

1/2 an avocado

1 banana

1 cup almond milk

1 teaspoon of chia seeds

1 tablespoon honey or maple syrup (optional)

Instruction:

1. Mix all the ingredients in a blender.

2. Blend until smooth.

3. Serve immediately.

4. Berry Lemonade

Ingredients:

1 cup of fresh or frozen berries (blueberries, raspberries, strawberries).

1/2 cup freshly squeezed lemon juice

4 cups of water

1/4 cup honey or maple syrup

Ice cubes

Lemon slices (for garnish)

Fresh mint leaves (for garnish)

Instruction:

1. Blend the blended berries and lemon juice in a blender until smooth.

2. Mix the berry mixture, water and honey in a jug. Mix well.

3. Serve over ice, garnished with lemon slices and fresh mint leaves.

5. Cucumber Mint Water

Ingredients:

1 cucumber, thinly sliced

1/4 cup fresh mint leaves

8 cups of water

Ice cubes

Instruction:

1. In a large pitcher, combine the cucumber slices, mint leaves, and water.

2. Refrigerate for at least two hours to let the flavors to blend.

3. Serve over ice.

www.ingramcontent.com/pod-product-compliance
Lightning Source LLC
Chambersburg PA
CBHW071024260726

48662CB00024B/1898